STRESS AND TIGER JUICE

STRESS AND TIGER JUICE

How to manage your stress and improve your life and your health

STEWART BEDFORD, PH.D.

SCOTT PUBLICATIONS

Chico, California

Published by:
    Scott Publications
    Post Office Box 3277
    Chico, CA 95927

Library of Congress Cataloging in Publication Data
Bedford, Stewart, 1980 —
    Stress and Tiger Juice:
    How to Manage Your Stress and Improve
    Your Life and Your Health

Bibliography: p. Includes index.
I. Stress (Psychology) 2. Stress (Physiology)
I. Title.
BF575.S75B35   158'.1   79-92277
ISBN 0-935930-00-0
ISBN 0-935930-01-9 pbk.

Dedicated to
    our children
    and grandchildren
    in the hope
    that future generations
    can have
    a clear view
    of the natural stress reaction
    in the human being.

Contents

Part Three — Stress of Stress Starts in Your Thinking and Can End There Too

Epilogue

Bibliography

Index

Preface

This book is designed to help you understand your stress reaction and learn to manage your deep emergency energy. It is not designed to give you instant happiness. It could increase your level of happiness, or at least reduce your unhappiness. It provides specific exercises you can use to regulate your stress reaction directly, through relaxation and meditation techniques. It also provides exercises to help you manage your stress at its source — in your thinking. It will show you how you may be making errors in thinking that cause you to waste stress energy, and it will show you ways of correcting errors of thinking so that you can improve your methods of stress management.

The book does not teach you how to change the things you think stress you — your stressors. It does deal with some of the ideas you have about your stressors. It is designed to help you learn ways to rethink some of these ideas so that you can manage your stress reactions at their source — in your thinking.

The exercises in the book are *simple*. They are not *easy*. If you are going to succeed with them, some practice will be necessary. When you do succeed, you will be more responsible for your own life. When you can manage your stress energies more efficiently, you will be better able to manage relationships, work, play, and your life in general.

In today's world there are many stressors. Vast quantities of tranquilizers are taken all over the world. Barrels of alcohol are consumed by people trying to cope. Other mind-altering chemicals are available on the street, in stores, and in offices. Many of these chemicals have unpleasant side-effects. The ideas in this book do not have unpleasant side-effects and they could help you reduce your intake of mind-altering chemicals if you rely on drugs to help you cope with your life and your stress reactions.

This book is not a "cure-all" for all of your problems. It *can* help you stop wasting stress hormones and help you conserve your deep emergency energy. It does describe alternatives open to you that you may not have realized were possible. Read the book, practice the exercises, and see what you can do with your life when you are in charge of you.

Acknowledgements

I am deeply grateful to all the people with whom I have worked in the past thirty years. The problems we have struggled with together have frequently been the result of stress, or at least have been aggravated by stress. This direct work with people has taught me much about stress and about people.

I am also grateful to the people who have done formal research on stress and stress management. I have given researchers and authors credit for their ideas and contributions and I have listed further reading in the Bibliography.

Some of the authors who have been particularly helpful to me have been: Herbert Benson, M.D.; Barbara Brown, Ph.D.; Walter Cannon, M.D.; Albert Ellis, Ph.D.; Maxie Maultsby, Jr., M.D.; Gary Schwartz, Ph.D.; and Hans Selye, M.D.

A special thanks goes to Sandy and Jim Rogers, Gary Bedford, Dwaine Jones, M.D., and Albert Raitt, Jr., M.D. for their critiques; Anne Blake for her critique and for excellent copy editing; Audy Van Ornum, my office manager and biofeedback assistant, for her typing and for her enthusiasm; Patti Goodwin-Walton for her proof-reading; Len Fulton for his invaluable consultation regarding publication; and Scott Bedford for promotion and business consultation.

Introduction

1

How to Use This Book

"The only thing we have to fear is fear itself." Franklin Delano Roosevelt said that in his first inaugural address, in 1933. During World War II he said it again. I heard him say it when I was a tailgunner on a B-24, flying combat over southern Europe. At the time, I was not reassured by my Commander In Chief. I thought I was afraid of Nazi fighter planes and antiaircraft flak.

Since World War II I have learned more technical things about fear. For over thirty years I have been doing psychotherapy with a wide variety of problems that people have faced. I have come to believe that President Roosevelt pointed out a very important thing to us, even though he overlooked fighter planes and flak. Fear is a part of our stress reaction and I am convinced that a great many human beings do have fear of fear. Others have anger about anger. Most of us do, indeed, get upset about being upset. We frequently do have "stress of stress." This book will help you reduce your upset feelings and it will help you manage your anger and fear more effectively.

When you get upset, you send signals from your brain to your body — signals that tell your body what to do to cope with emergencies. The signals are carried by nerve impulses and hormones, some of which come from a supply of deep emergency energy that you have. We don't know whether this hormone energy can be replenished when it is used. I think it cannot be replaced.

In this book, I will give you step-by-step ways that you can learn to manage and conserve your precious emergency energy.

You will learn that your stress reaction is natural, but that you can activate it by mistake. Some of your mistakes can be corrected by simple methods. Others will take more work on your part. The simple methods will teach you to manage your stress energy by changing your body signals. Methods of managing your body signals will be described in detail in Part Two of this book. The more complicated methods are described in Part Three. These methods will help you change the errors in your thinking that are causing you to send false alarm signals to your stress system.

You can start doing the exercises as you come to them in the book. Or, you can read the whole book and then go back to the exercises. I would suggest that you try the exercises as you go. The sooner you start, the sooner you will see some changes in your reactions. Whichever way you go, it is going to take practice. These methods are not magic.

The book includes some words from my imagination — "tiger juice" for example. I have also used the correct names for the things that happen to you when you stress yourself — "adrenocorticotrophic hormone" is a correct term, but "tiger juice" is easier for me to remember.

I have given researchers and authors credit for their ideas. When you see names and numbers in parentheses, look in the bibliography to find the source of the information and where you can read more about the ideas. Part One describes some of the research that has

14

been done on stress. It will give you technical information and can help you understand your own stress reaction.

One point I want to make loud and clear. This book is designed to help you *manage* your stress energy. It is not designed to prevent you from "having stress." Stress is a normal and helpful thing. You have stress when you are irritated. You have stress when you are in love. You can have it when you are excited and you can have it when you are bored. You need your stress energy to live. You will be more effective in your living when you improve your methods of stress management. If you are looking for quick and easy ways to prevent yourself from having stress, you may have to take medication. If you want to manage your stress energy in a natural way (and still have it available when you need it), read on.

A word of caution here. If you are taking medication (medication can be helpful), check with the doctor who prescribed it. If you are successful in doing the exercises in this book, you might need to reduce some medications. Tell your doctor that you are learning to do deep muscle relaxation. *Don't change your medication without talking to your doctor.*

This book is not intended as a substitute for medical treatment or counseling. It is a self-help book, but it is not self-analysis. The feedback you get from a professionally trained therapist can keep you focused on important areas of your problems. The book is not meant to substitute for therapy but it can supplement many forms of therapy. Discuss this with your therapist if you are getting help or thinking about getting help.

To help you use more brain power in managing your stress reaction, I have included "guided-imagery" exercises throughout the book. You see, your brain has two sides. Each side is a little different from the other, and each side can trigger your stress reaction. For example, as you read these words, the left half of your brain is processing the information (or, if you are in a small minority of people, the right half of your brain is processing the words for you). Since stress can be triggered by either side of your brain, I want you to start using *both* sides of your brain. Imagine that ideas are something like potatoes that have to be dug from the ground. After potatoes are dug, they are sorted in sacks and stored. In your mind's eye, visualize yourself digging potatoes, sorting them, sacking them, and storing them. When you are picturing yourself and potatoes in this manner, you are doing it with the right side of your brain (if you are in the majority of people). As you read on, you have other exercises for your right brain. Try them. They will help you manage your stress with both sides of your brain.

In addition to the right and left sides of your brain, you also have a conscious and a subconscious part of your mind. Since your subconscious mind can trigger your stress reaction too, you will manage your stress energy more effectively if you know more about the things that go on in the back of your mind — your subconscious. The last part of the book can help you understand what does go on in the back of your mind. You will learn how to be a better listener — when you are talking to yourself.

When I use the term "self-talk," I am talking about the way you think — the way you interpret events, situations, scenes, reactions and things. These interpretations, often subconscious, can influence the way you use your stress energy. Epictetus, a Stoic philosopher,

16

described this process when he said, "People feel disturbed, not by things, but by the views which they take of things." (Epictetus lived almost two thousand years ago and he was at one time a slave. He spoke with the language of his time and he knew a lot about stress.)

Learn what stress is all about in Part One of this book. In Part Two, learn how to manage your stress reaction directly. In Part Three, learn how to prevent your thinking from triggering your stress reaction in error.

Part One
Stress is Natural

2

In the Beginning — A History of Stress

A long time ago, Saber Tooth Tigers were alive and well. They had two front teeth that were mean tools, and they ate meat. They were probably tough customers — especially when they were hungry.

Fossil bones have led scientists to believe that some of our ancestors were also alive and well when Saber Tooth Tigers were around. We may have friendly feelings towards our ancestors, but the tigers saw them mainly as meat. I suspect that our ancestors did not like the idea of being seen mainly as meat. They were probably willing to run fast or fight hard — to keep from being mainly meat.

It would seem possible that some of our ancestors were better than others at fighting or getting away from the tigers (as well as other hungry creatures). I believe that our ancestors who were better at fighting and running passed their skills and systems on to their children and grandchildren. Some people call this the "survival of the fittest." That's the way nature works.

One of the systems that was passed on is now called the "fight-or-flight reaction." This reaction is a type of emergency system. It was undoubtedly a big help to our ancestors who did not want to be lunch for Saber Tooth Tigers. When they used their emergency reactions, they could fight harder or run faster than they could without the reaction. They probably welcomed all the help they could get when they were running from or fighting tigers. They needed their fight-or-flight reactions to survive.

How did our ancestors get help from their emergency reactions? First of all, they got electrical and chemical messages that were sent from their brains to various parts of their bodies. Some of the electrical messages were nerve signals that went from their brains to their muscles. The signals told the muscles what to do in fleeing or fighting. Some of the chemical messengers started in the part of our ancestors' brains called the hypothalamus. These messengers signaled pituitary glands which in turn signaled adrenal glands. The adrenal glands put special hormones into the blood streams of our ancient relatives. These signals must have helped our ancestors survive — or how else would we be alive and well ourselves?

Here are some of the things the electrical and chemical signals started in our ancestors' bodies. Muscles were tensed so they could move faster and fight better. Hearts were speeded up to pump more blood and deliver more energy and oxygen. Breathing was accelerated to capture more oxygen and to get rid of carbon dioxide. Digestion was slowed down or stopped. Tiny blood vessels at skin level contracted so that blood was shunted to parts of the body which were needed for fighting or fleeing — parts such as the large muscles, the heart, and the lungs. (This gave our ancestors more strength and may have resulted in less blood loss in case they were bitten or scratched by tigers.) Muscles that controlled bowels and bladders relaxed so that excess baggage could be dumped (no need to carry that stuff around for long runs or tough fights).

These are a few of the important things that happened when primitive people were in danger from stressors they faced. We don't know what the people called these systems. We can guess that they were glad the systems were working. At least they were probably glad when they could outrun or outfight the cats with the two long teeth.

3
Stress Today

There aren't too many Saber Tooth Tigers around today. We don't have to run or fight as much as our ancestors did. We still have danger, though, and we have to run fast sometimes. We may even have to fight occasionally if we want to survive. When we do need to run fast or fight hard, it is still handy to have extra energy. Once in a while we need our stress reactions to survive physical danger.

Today we live in a different world than our ancestors did. Our jungles are asphalt and many of our tigers are paper — stacks and stacks of paper. We live in a complex world. We have many pressures. We have payments to make, forms to fill, signs to read, taxes to pay, laws to obey, and deadlines to meet. We worry a lot.

Most of our worries involve thinking and planning and talking and writing. These things take energy, but not the intense, short-term energy our emergency systems provide (scientists believe that the fight-or-flight reaction was meant to be used for only a few minutes at a time). Unfortunately, many of us start our emergency systems going with our worries. It's as though the old part of our brain — the hypothalamus — doesn't know the difference between paper tigers and real tigers. When we worry, we can (and often do) start stress reactions going. Then we keep the stress reactions going for long periods of time. We don't use the stress energy by running or fighting, so we build up tension and conflict in our systems. On the one hand we are triggering the stress reaction to get us going, and on the other hand we are trying to remain cool, calm, and collected in order to think ourselves out of our worries.

It would be helpful to us to remember that our stress reactions are basically the same as those of our ancient ancestors. Our worries are different than theirs, but our reactions are the same. When they reacted to tigers, they got help. When we react in the same way to paper tigers, we can get sick. Also, keep in mind that our reactions are natural, and that we all have them, even though some of us may react more strongly than others.

To show how this works, let's try a little experiment. First, get yourself relaxed and comfortable. Slow down your system and ease yourself into your favorite place to relax. Now, imagine yourself walking in some quiet woods. It's morning and a beautiful day. You've had breakfast and you feel great. You are walking along and all you have with you is a stout walking stick. You are relaxed. You are glad to be alive. Think about this until you can experience some of the pleasant feelings.

Now, in your imagination, walk on a little further. Imagine walking around a clump of bushes and coming face to face with a wild creature that has a mean and hungry look about it. Let your body react as it probably would if this really happened to you. For a moment, let your body experience what it would be like to be eyeball-to-eyeball with a creature that wanted to kill you. Get in touch with your emergency energy. Feel your

26

fight-or-flight reaction. Get to know your stress as nature intended you to know it — when you have to run or fight to survive.

Did you feel your muscles tense? Did you feel a catch in your throat? Did you grip your walking stick with cold, sweaty hands? Did your digestion stop and your stomach flutter? Did you feel any urge to go to the toilet? Did your heart pound? Did you breathe faster? Did you feel dizzy? Did you feel any impulse to run or fight? If you allowed your imagination to go with the fantasy, you may have experienced some of these things.

You see, if you really did have to face down a tiger, you would want to have these things happen. You would be more likely to survive if they did happen. If they were happening, nature would be programming you in ways that would be helpful to you — and you would probably welcome all the help you could get. If you felt tense, your large muscles were getting ready to help you run or fight. If your hands started to sweat, it was to help you cool off as you ran or fought. If you felt your stomach flutter, it was the blood being directed away from your intestines. If you felt the urge to go to the toilet, chemicals were relaxing muscles that controlled your lower intestinal tract. If your heart started to pound, it was trying to get more blood to your larger muscle groups. If your breathing rate increased, it was to get more oxygen around in your body. If you felt dizzy, blood was being diverted away from your brain to other parts of your body.

Now, relax again. We'll do another guided fantasy. This time, put yourself in a place in your everyday life where you sometimes experience emotional upsets. Only you can know where this is and what usually happens. Again, it is a nice day and you feel good when you first start the fantasy. You are at ease and you feel relaxed. Relax and think about your world.

Think about a recent time when you were upset. In your mind's eye, act out the scene again. Have other people do what they did when you stressed yourself. Imagine yourself feeling upset as you did when it happened. Allow your body to respond as it usually does when this happens. Experience your stress reaction in your world. Compare your stress reaction in your world to the stress reaction you experienced when you were out in the fantasy jungle facing down a mean and hungry animal.

Now, relax again and think about what happened in your world. Did you experience any of the same things you did with your wild creature? Did your muscles tense? Did you feel a catch in your throat? Did your hands feel cold and sweaty? Did your digestion stop? Did you feel any urge to go to the toilet? Did your breathing change? Did your heart pound? Did you feel any impulse to run or fight? Did you experience any of your fight-or-flight reaction?

Think about your own situation. How much good does physical fighting and physical escaping do in solving the problems you face in your complex world? It may be that you need extreme physical exertion to handle your emergencies, but then again, maybe you don't. Please understand, I believe that physical exercise is an important part of a stress management program (see Chapter Eight, Exercise), but it could be that you are programming more of your stress reaction than you need for emergencies that do not require fighting or fleeing. It could be that you are over-reacting to your day-to-day pressures — your stressors. If you don't face physical danger, your own stress reaction could be a danger itself!

Your stress reaction, triggered in error for any length of time, could be detrimental to your health.

When we trigger our stress reactions in error, we can program ourselves into full-scale stress reactions. We can go from irritation, to anger, all the way into fury. We can go from a little nervousness, to anxiety, on into complete panic. We can worry ourselves into having ulcers, high blood pressure, headaches, heart attacks, or worse yet, cold, sweaty hands when we are trying to impress friends or clients. If you want to prevent some of these things from happening to you, read on and learn ways you can keep yourself from triggering your stress reaction in error.

4

Stress of Stress — Errors in Signaling

How do we make errors in our signaling systems? How do we start our fight-or-flight reactions going when we are *not* faced with danger? We do it with our thinking. We think our bodies are in danger. We do this sometimes when there aren't any tigers around. We imagine that we are in physical danger when we are in psychological danger. When this happens, we are usually worried about what other people think of us. We picture ourselves as being seen as dumb, foolish, weak, chicken, and other things we don't like. Usually, we don't want other people to think of us as dumb, foolish, weak, chicken, or any of these other things. We want them to have better pictures of us in their heads. We want them to have images we like. Sometimes, we get images mixed up with bodies. We think our image is being destroyed in the minds of people. Even if that is true, our bodies are usually safe. Safe from danger outside — not necessarily from inside. When we think our image is being destroyed, the part of our brain called the hypothalamus can trigger our stress reactions in error. The error is that we don't need to run or fight to survive.

For example, suppose you have to talk to a group of people and you feel nervous and tense. Maybe you aren't quite as tense as you would be if you were facing a hungry tiger, but then again, you could be even more nervous. What you are doing is signaling danger and getting ready to run or fight when all you are planning to do is talk. When this happens, the ideas in your head are scaring your hypothalamus. Your hypothalamus is then getting you in gear to save your life. You are sending false alarm messages around in your body and these false alarms are the errors in signaling that leave you feeling upset.

You see, the older part of your brain (your hypothalamus) doesn't know the difference between hungry tigers and people in audiences. What you may be thinking to yourself is, "I wonder what these people really think of me. Wouldn't it be horrible if they thought I was stupid!" In this way, you may be concerned about your image. You don't want the people in the audience to have negative images of you. If you think the images they have are different from the ones you want them to have, you could scare your hypothalamus into thinking you are in danger. This might in turn get your body ready to survive that danger and to defend itself by either running or fighting.

Some of us create even more stress in our systems when we are trying to control our stress reactions. What we sometimes do is try to brace ourselves so that our stress reactions don't show. In this process, we can actually increase our stress reactions. We can have fear about our fear, anger about our anger, and upset about our upsets. I call this *"stress of stress."*

Let me give you an example from my own experience. Once, when I was younger, I was reading a paper to some professional people in the mental health field. Some of these people were well known and most of them had written and read many papers themselves. I was standing on a small platform, talking into a microphone. When I started to talk, I realized that my knees were shaking. I got concerned and said to myself, "What will these experts think of me? Here I am, reading a paper about nervousness, and I'm nervous. This is horrible!"

As I stood there, a brilliant idea occurred to me. I said to myself, "Lock your knees, dummy, then you won't shake."

Unfortunately, I listened to myself. I did just that. I braced myself and locked my knees tight. Then, a short time later, I realized that my whole body was shaking. Somehow I managed to finish the paper before the vicious cycle shook me off the platform. I was without a doubt experiencing stress of stress.

Later, as I went back over the experience in fantasy, I learned a lot about myself and my inner messages. I learned how I had been thinking myself into sending false alarm messages around in my body. Some of my thoughts were, "People out there may think this is a stupid paper. Then they will think I am stupid. It will be horrible if they think I am stupid." About that time, the old part of my brain read this as a danger signal and started flashing "run" signals through my body. My legs got the message to run and carry my body out of the danger area. At the same time, in another part of my brain, I was thinking, "If you run out of here, they will *really* think you are stupid. On top of that, they will know that you know you are stupid, and that will be even more horrible. Don't run, dummy, brace yourself and go on reading your paper."

As you can see, I had two sets of messages going in the subconscious part of my mind. One was telling me to run, and the other was telling me to brace myself. My muscles didn't know what to do so they tried to do both at the same time. That's how my knees started to shake. If I had told my muscles to relax, I wouldn't have started the vicious cycle going. (Better yet, if I hadn't scared myself with my own errors in thinking, I wouldn't have been in trouble in the first place.)

In Part Two of this book, I will tell you about some ways of learning to control what your body does when you trigger your stress reaction in error. In Part Three, we will go into detail about ways in which you may be thinking yourself into unnecessary stress. We will consider new ways of thinking — ways that may prevent you from triggering tiger juice when there aren't any tigers around. Before we do that, however, we will consider some of the more technical aspects of stress. The next chapter will tell you more about tiger juice and what it really is.

5

Anatomy of Stress — What is Tiger Juice?

The stress reaction is natural, therefore the things that happen in our bodies when we have stress are also natural. Our ancestors survived Saber Tooth Tigers because they had stress reactions that furnished them with emergency energy. I call this energy "tiger juice" to remind me of its natural purpose — to help me run from or fight tigers. That way, I can remind myself to conserve the special energy when I am upset and there aren't any tigers around.

Research has not come up with a clear answer about the amount of tiger juice we have. Some people believe that we have a fixed amount and that when it's gone, it's gone. Other people believe we can replenish the deep energies of the stress reaction just as we can replenish our more superficial reserve energy. Since I don't know for sure, I want to conserve my stress energies as much as possible. Calling the energy "tiger juice" has helped me conserve my energy and has also helped people I have trained in stress management.

When I use the term "tiger juice," I'm talking about two kinds of "juice" — the electrical messengers of nerve signals and the chemical messengers of our hormones. When you read the technical names of these messengers, you may also wish to call them "tiger juice." If the term helps you remember the real and natural purposes of your stress reaction, I'm glad. It could help you survive with less stress of stress. It could help you save your stress energies for real tigers.

Many scientists have studied our stress reactions and the emergency energy we all have. A great deal of careful research has been done on tiger juice — even if the scientists haven't used that term. Here is a short summary of some of the research.

Walter Cannon, a physiologist at the University of Chicago, did early research on stress (6). He studied cats. Dr. Cannon described cats' reaction to danger. He listed the physiological changes in the cats when they were confronted with danger—mostly dogs. He called their reaction the fight-or-flight response. This response has apparently been around for a long time, and the human being has a response pattern that is very similar to other creatures, including cats.

Hans Selye (27), an endocrinologist, is also a well-known expert on stress. Dr. Selye has written many books on stress and he is president of the International Institute of Stress. Dr. Selye has described a series of events that take place in us when we are in trouble. He calls it the General Adaptation Syndrome (G.A.S.). Dr. Selye has done a great deal of research and has expanded the work done by Dr. Cannon. He has shown that there are three stages in our general adaptation syndromes. The first he calls the alarm reaction; the second, the stage of resistance; and the third, the stage of exhaustion.

The general alarm is similar to the fight-or-flight reaction. It includes most of the physiological events described by Dr. Cannon in his work.

The stage of resistance comes after the alarm reaction stops and the creature starts adapting to the stressors it faces. In this stage, resistance goes up and the creature tries to cope with whatever is wrong.

The stage of exhaustion follows severe stress that lasts for a long time. In this stage, the symptoms of the alarm reaction come back and are usually irreversible. In this stage, the creature often dies.

The fight-or-flight alarm reaction begins in the part of the brain called the hypothalamus. This is a small part of the brain, bigger than a bean, but smaller than a prune. It's the boss of the autonomic nervous system and it triggers the adrenal glands which in turn shoot chemicals, or hormones, into our blood streams when we are in danger. Two of these hormones are epinephrine and norepinephrine. These hormones work as messengers that tell parts of our body to do things—things that help us in emergencies. These chemicals activate our autonomic nervous systems and our autonomic systems play an important part in our stress reactions. When we run into tigers, we really do get extra "juice" when we need to fight tigers or run from them. We need our "tiger juice" when we meet tigers!

When we are in danger, our muscles tense up from messages sent by our autonomic nerves. Then, chemicals get into our blood stream and reinforce some of the things that are starting to happen. A few of the things that happen are: our blood pressure goes up; the tiny vessels at skin level constrict so that our hands and feet feel cold; digestion stops so that we feel like we have butterflies in our stomach; we get an increase in perspiration which we call "cold sweat"; and the muscles that control our bladder and bowels relax so that we feel a need to go to the toilet.

Other things that happen are: the spleen releases more red corpuscles to carry oxygen; the bone marrow starts making white corpuscles faster; and the liver is stimulated to produce more sugar. When the hypothalamus starts the reaction, it stimulates the pituitary glands. Then two more chemicals get into the act, the thyrotrophic hormone (TTH) and the adrenocorticotrophic hormone (ACTH). TTH stimulates the thyroid which in turn regulates body metabolism. ACTH starts other chemicals flowing from the adrenal cortex.

All these messages, nerve and chemical, get us geared up to fight or run so that we can survive against physical danger. When we have to fight or run to survive, all of these things are handy to have. We need our stress reactions to stay alive when we face danger.

Dr. Walter Hess (11), a physiologist and Nobel Prize winner, also did research on cats. He showed that stimulation of a cat's hypothalamus produced the changes that we can see in the fight-or-flight reaction. He also found that stimulation of another part of the cat's hypothalamus produced changes that seemed to be the opposite of the fight-or-flight reaction. This was a reaction that seemed to start relaxation going in the cats. He called this the trophotropic response. He thought the purpose of the response was for protection against "overstress."

Dr. Herbert Benson, author of the best-selling book, *The Relaxation Response* (3), did extensive research to show that human beings are as smart as cats and that we also have a trophotropic response. Dr. Benson calls ours the "relaxation response." He studied several methods of relaxation and meditation and showed that the physiological changes are about the same for the various methods. He also proved that human beings can learn to control their stress reactions.

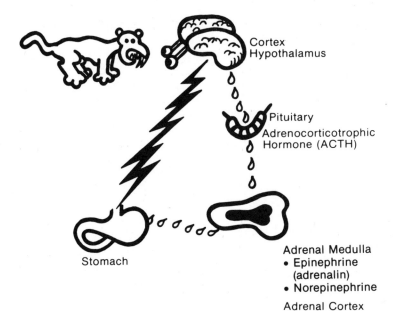

Cortex
Hypothalamus

Pituitary
Adrenocorticotrophic
Hormone (ACTH)

Stomach

Adrenal Medulla
- Epinephrine
  (adrenalin)
- Norepinephrine

Adrenal Cortex
- Corticoids

Anatomy
of *STRESS*
and
TIGER JUICE

As you can see, there are some long, technical names in the anatomy of stress. That is why I use the term "tiger juice." It's much easier for me to remember than adrenocorticotrophic hormone—and adrenocorticotrophic hormone is just one of the juices.

Now you know a few things about your stress reaction. The rest of the book will show you ways you can manage your tiger juice — hopefully with more fun and with less stress of stress.

Part Two
Stress Energy
Can Be Managed

6
Relaxation

It is hard to be tense and relaxed at the same time. If you want to learn a natural way of managing your stress reaction, learn to relax. Research has shown that deep muscle relaxation is one way you can manage your body's stress energy. This chapter will teach you a form of deep muscle relaxation. Learn to do it. Practice it. Relaxation is a very important part of some of the other things you will be learning later on in this book.

You can follow these instructions by yourself, or you can have a friend read them to you. You could even read the instructions to a tape recorder and then listen to yourself. Either way, you can learn the technique. When you learn it, you won't have to depend on your friend or your tape. You will know the method.

First, find a comfortable place to relax. You can do it lying down on a bed or the floor. You can do it in a recliner or sitting in a chair. If you practice relaxing in different places and in different positions, it will be easier for you to transfer this training into your life in general. After you have learned to relax, you will probably want to relax in more than one way and in more than one place. If you relax sitting down, it will be easier to relax while sitting at your desk or driving your car. If you relax while lying down, it will be easier to learn to go to sleep when you want to.

Don't wear shoes or tight clothes or tight jewelry. It's best to be warm, but not too hot.

When you get yourself into a comfortable position, take a deep breath. Fill your lungs with air while you count slowly to ten. Then let the air out—all out. Concentrate on how your lungs feel when they are full of air and how they feel when they are empty.

Now think about your hands. Tense the muscles in your hands. Make fists. Think about how your hands feel when they are tense. Hold the tension while you count slowly to ten. Now relax the muscles in your hands and think about how they feel when they are relaxed. Concentrate on how your hands feel.

Now tense the muscles in your shoulders and arms. Think about how these muscles feel when they are tense. Hold this tension while you count slowly to ten. Now relax and think about how the muscles feel when they are relaxed. Get acquainted with your tense feelings. Get acquainted with your relaxed feelings. Learn how your body feels.

Now tense the muscles in your forehead. Raise your eyebrows as high as you can and think about how your face feels (think about how your face *feels*, not how it looks). Count slowly to ten and then relax. Now think about how these muscles feel when they are relaxed. Remember, think about the muscles when they are tense and when they are relaxed.

Now tense the muscles in your jaws. Clamp your teeth together and concentrate on how the muscles feel. Count slowly to ten and then relax. Now think about the muscles in your jaws when they are relaxed.

Take another deep breath. Hold the air in while you count slowly to ten. Think about your chest. Let the air out slowly and relax. Think about your chest when it is relaxed.

Arch your back a little and tense your back muscles. Hold the tension and think about it while you count slowly to ten. Now relax and think about the back muscles when they are relaxed.

Tighten the muscles in your stomach. Pretend that someone is going to sock you with a medicine ball and you are going to brace yourself so it doesn't hurt. Concentrate on the tight muscles. Count slowly to ten. Relax. Think about the muscles in your stomach when they are relaxed.

Tense the muscles in both legs and both feet. Hold the tension while you count slowly to ten. Think about the muscles when they are tense. Relax. Now think about the muscles when they are relaxed.

Now, try to relax all the muscles in your body. Get as comfortable as you can. Concentrate on your breathing. Think about the air coming into your body and going out of your body. Air coming in. Air going out. Concentrate on your breathing. Breathe deeply. Breathe slowly. Practice letting your stomach muscles pull the air in and push the air out. Concentrate on this and do this kind of breathing for about five minutes. If you start thinking about other ideas, pull your thoughts back to your breathing. Air coming in. Air going out. Air coming in. Air going out.

If you go to sleep while doing this part of the exercise, don't worry. If you stay awake, you will get more good out of the relaxation, but a little sleep doesn't hurt us now and then. If you do these exercises twice a day, you will gradually learn how to get into deep muscle relaxation. When you have learned to control relaxation in your muscles, you have learned one of the methods of managing your stress energies. You have learned a little more about the control of your emergency reaction. Remember, it is hard to be tense and relaxed at the same time.

Some of these instructions are modifications of Progressive Relaxation, a system developed by Dr. Edmund Jacobson (14).

Mini-methods of Relaxation

If you have a busy life style, you may not be able to do twenty minutes of relaxation twice a day. You would be more healthy if you did, but if you can't, learn to do mini-exercises when you can. Five minutes relaxation is better than none. Twenty seconds relaxation is also better than none. Practice relaxing your muscles when you have to wait. When you stop at a stop sign, take a deep breath and relax your muscles while you count slowly to ten. Get into the habit. Learn to do it automatically. You will arrive at your destination with less tension. You will drive more efficiently if you relax when you can.

If you are used to making telephone calls under pressure, take ten seconds to relax between calls. When you start to hang up, hold the phone over the phone cradle while you take a deep breath, relax, and count slowly to ten. You won't get another call until you hang up. You will be more effective in your next call if you turn down your stress reaction. (Remember, you are trying to *manage* your stress reaction, not trying to turn it off completely.)

Are you a clock watcher? Every time you look at a clock or watch, remind yourself to relax. Each time you look, take a deep breath and count slowly to ten. If you reduce your stress reaction, you will probably worry less about time and increase your efficiency. That way, you can easily spare ten seconds now and then. If you learn to do this regularly, you will be surprised what it does for your health.

Another simple method of stress management involves control of breathing — Dr. Maxie Maultsby (17) calls this "Instant Sanity." I like the method. It has helped me and many people with whom I have worked. To do it, you take a deep breath and then exhale all the air you can. Then you wait at least ten seconds before breathing in again. As you practice this method, try to extend the number of seconds you wait before breathing in again. Learn to do this exercise. At first, you can practice during television commercials. After you have learned how the exercise is done, you can do it almost anywhere without other people knowing what you are doing.

Again, it is hard to be relaxed and tense at the same time. Practice these relaxation procedures and learn to control your muscles. Your stress management will improve when you do.

7

Meditation

Meditation can be helpful in the management of your natural emergency reaction. It can help you control your fight-or-flight response. It can help you regulate your tiger juice and save your stress energy for real live tigers. Most people who meditate every day have less trouble with health problems related to stress (heart attacks, high blood pressure, ulcers, colitis, backaches, and headaches, just to mention a few).

I will describe some techniques of meditation I use in stress management. I use them myself in my own stress management and I teach them to others in my work. The methods involve concentration. If you did the relaxation exercises in Chapter Six, you have done one form of meditation. When you focused your attention on your breathing, you were doing a form of meditation that has been around for centuries. It works.

The methods of meditation I am going to describe can be added to the one you learned in Chapter Six. Read this (Chapter Seven), and then try the methods that sound interesting to you. I believe you can have fun while you are meditating.

Current research suggests that parts of our brains have special functions. For most of us, the left side of our brain thinks in words and abstract ideas. The right side of our brain thinks in images. Dr. Gary Schwartz (26), believes that some types of meditation work better for the left side of our brain and some work better for the right side. Most forms of meditation slow down our stress reactions, while other methods seem to go further than that, and quiet our minds. Some methods work for some people and not for others. You will have to be the judge as to what works best for you.

Like relaxation, meditation can be done in different positions. I suggest that you practice the various methods of meditation described, and that you do them in positions that are easy for you. Remember, it is going to be important for you to transfer your skills in meditation and relaxation to your life in general. You will not always be able to sit or lie in one position. Try these exercises in different ways.

It will be easier to stay awake if you are sitting rather than lying down. But again, sleep is not all that bad — unless you are driving a car or other vehicle. (Do not practice these exercises while you are driving or while you are in dangerous situations.)

Breathing Meditation

When you relax your muscles and concentrate your attention on your breathing, you are meditating. As you do it, you are probably changing some of your body functions. It is a good basic method to use in stress management. You will have to practice for a long time before you can keep your mind off other things during your meditation. Don't worry about it. When other ideas come to mind, pull your attention back to your breathing. Think about the air coming into your body. Think about the air going out of your body. Put other ideas on hold, or let them just pass quietly through your mind. Then, pull your attention back to your breathing.

Mantra Meditation

A mantra can be a short phrase, a prayer, a word, or a repetitive sound that you make. Some groups have suggested strict secrecy of mantras and have made claims that the "power" of the mantra is lost if it is revealed to others. I think that is nonsense. The power of meditation is in the processs, not in the props.

If you have a mantra that works for you, use it. If you don't, make one up. Try a special word you like to say — I had fun and success with "flamingo."

Some people believe that words with "m" and "n" work best. They may be right. Many mantras from the past have had these sounds. If you can't think of a word, try the age-old mantra "om." When you do, hold the "mmm" sound as you think it to yourself.

Prayers have made great mantras for thousands of years. Dr. Herbert Benson (3) says that nearly all cultures and religions have procedures that incorporate meditation and the whole relaxation response. He believes that meditation is no more dangerous to people than prayers. I agree.

When you have picked (or been assigned) a mantra, relax your muscles and think about it. Repeat it over and over to yourself. You can say it out loud, but most people don't. Just think it to yourself. When other ideas come to mind, pull your attention gently back to your mantra. Try it (along with the relaxation) for two twenty-minute periods each day. I like to do it early in the morning before breakfast and late in the afternoon before my evening meal. See what time is best for you.

Visualization Meditation

You can meditate by concentrating your attention on some object. You can also meditate by closing your eyes and creating an image of an object in your mind's eye. I would suggest you try it with your eyes closed. If you do, it will help you with the exercises in Chapter Ten (Desensitization).

Think of something you like to look at. A flower, a simple scene, a candle, or a piece of sculpture. Form an image in your mind's eye. Keep your attention on the image. Again, when other ideas come to mind, pull your attention gently back to your image. Relax. Enjoy your picture.

You may have trouble getting a clear picture at first. Try looking at a picture or object for a minute or two. Then, close your eyes and try to hold the picture in your mind's eye as long as you can. With practice you will increase your ability. If you want more information about this interesting technique, read Mike and Nancy Samuels' magnificent book, *Seeing With the Mind's Eye: The History, Techniques and Uses of Visualization* (24).

There are other methods of meditation. I have listed several good books in the bibliography. Keep in mind that mantra meditation quiets the left brain, while visualization quiets the right brain. That's enough reason to know more than one method.

A word or two about the time it takes to meditate. I found that trading twenty minutes of sleep in the morning and twenty minutes of sleep in the evening was well worth it. When I started doing meditation regularly, I found that I slept more soundly when I did sleep and that I got to sleep easier than before. I also felt more rested and full of energy throughout the day. That's a fair trade. Find the time and meditate. You will be happy with the results.

8

Exercise

How much of the oxygen you breathe do you really use? The more efficient you are at processing oxygen, the more reserve energy you have. The more reserve energy you have, the better you are going to be at managing your stress system.

You don't have much reserve energy if you feel tired just walking around doing the minimum things you do to survive. If your reserve energy is low, you may be using much more of your tiger juice than you need to. And remember, we don't know whether your deep-level emergency energy (tiger juice) can be replenished when it's gone. We know you can replace your reserve energy without much trouble, *if you have a good working system for processing oxygen*.

Regular exercise can increase your efficiency in processing oxygen. Therefore, regular exercise plays a very important part in stress management.

Your delivery system for oxygen depends on several things: the strength of your pump and the amount of blood it can pump per stroke; the size and condition of your hoses; and the amount of blood you have. You can strengthen your system with exercise. If you have a strong oxygen-delivery system you will have more reserve energy. You won't be using as much of your deep reserve energies.

Another way in which exercise can be helpful in stress management has to do with self-image. If you are healthy and reasonably strong, chances are you have a better self-image than you would if you were weak and run-down. The stronger your self-image, the less vulnerable you feel. In other words, the better you feel about yourself, the better you can handle frustration and cope with the stressors in your life. Exercise usually helps build self-confidence — an important ingredient in feeling better about oneself.

Exercise can also be used directly to work off the energies of stress when you do overreact to a situation that does not require physical effort to survive. If you trigger your fight-or-flight reaction in error, you would probably feel more comfortable if you did get some exercise immediately.

There are some problems, however, with having exercise as the only means of handling the energies of stress triggered in error. For example, you may not always be able to work off the extra energy. Your boss would probably not understand if you insisted on running in place every time you upset yourself on your job.

How much regular exercise are you getting? Is exercise a part of your system of stress management? If you are not getting much exercise, and you really want to improve your stress management, start doing some planning about an exercise program for yourself. A good place to start is with your doctor. Find out what kind of shape you are in and get expert advice about a starting point and any special problems you may have. Running, walking, swimming, and biking are all good exercise to increase your efficiency in breathing and circulating blood. However, each person is an individual, and what is good for one may not be good for another. Get a good physical examination and talk about an exercise program with your doctor. *Then start doing it.* Talking will not be enough exercise to increase your reserve energies.

After you know about your own physical condition, you have many options. You can sign up for some exercise program. You can buy all kinds of exercise equipment, or you can get a good book and follow the plans outlined. Three excellent books are: *The New Aerobics*, by Dr. Kenneth Cooper, (7); *Total Fitness in 30 Minutes a Week*, by Laurence Morehouse and Leonard Gross, (19); and, *Doctor Solomon's Proven Master Plan For Total Body Fitness and Maintenance*, by Neil Solomon and Evalee Harrison, (30).

After you have your exercise system going, you can include some of the things I have suggested before. For example, exercise and increase your heart rate. Then see how fast you can reduce it again by relaxation. The better you are able to do that, the more efficient you are going to be at managing your stress reaction.

With practice, you could learn to do some meditation procedures along with your exercise. Make sure you are doing your exercises in a safe place, however. Do not try to meditate while you are running in places that have heavy traffic.

Techniques of this type have been taught to Olympic athletes. If the methods can help highly skilled athletes, they could also help you and me. Have fun. Exercise and meditate your way into better stress management.

9

Biofeedback

Have you used a biofeedback instrument today? Think. Biofeedback has been around since primitive people looked at their reflections in quiet ponds or streams. When was the last time you looked in a mirror? Other biofeedback devices have also been around for a long time. How long has it been since you weighed yourself?

Biofeedback gives you information about yourself and your body—information you can use to understand or change yourself. Most biofeedback instruments are more complicated than mirrors and scales. Today's biofeedback instruments can measure: the amount you sweat; your skin temperature; the amount of tension in your muscles; or the strength of brain waves in your head. When you get this type of information fed back to you, you can learn to control what your body does. You can learn to control functions in ways you may have thought impossible.

So what does all this have to do with stress? A lot, really. When you can raise your hand temperature, reduce your sweating, relax your muscles, and control your brain waves, you have reduced the stress chemicals in your blood stream and the tension in your system. You have learned to manage your stress energy.

Actually, you can learn to control stress without biofeedback. However, biofeedback instruments can help you learn much faster and with more accuracy. For example, it is hard to tell how much tension you have in your forehead muscles. Relax them now. Get the muscles as relaxed as you can. Do you have 10 or 50 microvolts of electricity going from your brain, down your motor nerves to your muscles? A microvolt is one millionth of a volt, so either way, it's not very much juice. You could, however, have enough tension to cause you trouble, even when you were as relaxed as you thought you could get. With a biofeedback instrument that measures muscle tension, you could learn to tell the difference between 10 microvolts and 50 microvolts of muscle tension. When you know that difference, you can be more sure of your relaxation methods. To do this, you would need to consult someone in the health professions who has been trained in the science of biofeedback.

Biofeedback Experiment

Would you like to try a little biofeedback experiment? Get a thermometer. A small weather thermometer will do (the kind you put in your mouth to measure body temperature won't work—most of them don't have enough range). An indoor-outdoor type thermometer will work. Color photography thermometers are great.

First, take your hand temperature. Hold the thermometer lightly between your thumb and forefinger. Wait about a minute—or until the liquid in the thermometer stops moving. Then, write down the temperature so you can remember it. Now, do the relaxation exercises in Chapter Six.

After you have done the relaxation exercises, take your hand temperature again and write it down. Did it go up? If it did, you probably reduced the stress chemicals in your blood stream. You controlled your tiger juice! (If your hand temperature was close to body temperature to begin with, it probably didn't go up much—you may not have had much stress chemical in your blood stream.) Remember, skin temperature can vary quite a bit even though your body temperature stays close to 98.6 degrees Fahrenheit, or 37.1 degrees Celsius. When you raise your hand temperature by relaxing, you are reducing the chemicals in your blood stream that cause the smooth muscles in the tiny arterials to contract. That reduces the amount of blood flowing through the vessels at skin level so the temperature in your skin goes down. In a remote way, your thermometer can be a gauge of how much tiger juice you are pumping.

Step by step, this is the way it works. Somewhere in your mind you decide to tense or relax your muscles. You send messages from the outer part of your brain, your cerebral cortex, to your muscles, telling them what to do. These messages travel down your motor nerves in a way that is like electrical energy going down a wire. If you want to tense your muscles, you zap them with more electrical energy. If you want to relax your muscles, you reduce the amount of electrical energy. When you relax your muscles, the hypothalamus seems to read this as an all-clear signal and sends messages to reduce the stress hormones—tiger juice—in your blood stream. When the stress chemicals are reduced, the smooth muscles in your arterials allow the vessels to enlarge. When the vessels enlarge, you have more blood flowing through them and your skin temperature goes up. In this way, you can decide to raise or lower your hand temperature. You can decide to control your stress energy. Remember, though, it will take a lot of practice before you're able to do this quickly.

If you are having a lot of stress, your hand temperature could be less than 70 degrees Fahrenheit, or 20 degrees Celsius. If you don't have much stress chemical in your blood stream, your hand temperature will be just a little below body temperature.

After you have practiced relaxation and have recorded your hand temperature a number of times, you will get good at guessing. You will have incorporated a biofeedback method into your own system.

Try another experiment. Take your thermometer with you wherever you go. When you think you are experiencing some stress, take your hand temperature. If your hand temperature is low, try to relax. See if you can raise your hand temperature right on the spot. (If you are having stress because you are running from a tiger, forget it. Nature knows best when it comes to real tigers.)

Keep in mind that hand temperature is just one of the things you can change when you are into your stress reaction (when your blood runs cold). In your fight-or-flight reaction, your rectal and bladder sphincters can try to open (when you have the you-know-what scared out of you). Your digestion can be interrupted (you have butterflies in your stomach). You can sweat a lot (the cold sweats). Even your hair can react (you can bristle with anger).

When you change your hand temperature, you are probably changing other things in your body. These are things you need to have happen when you deal with tigers—things you do not need to have happen when you deal with bosses, employees, teachers, students, parents, kids, doctors, patients, and clients, and friends, and relatives. You do need some of your stress energy to deal with these non-tigers, but it is important to learn to manage the stress reaction so that you don't waste stress energy and end up with stress of stress. Your biofeedback systems can help you in this respect.

10

Imagination and Desensitization

By now, if you have been practicing, you are probably getting good at relaxing your muscles. You may also be able to concentrate your attention and to meditate. If you can do these things, you are learning to manage your stress reaction. If you do the exercises regularly, you also have a method of keeping your stress down between exercises. The next problem is trying to transfer this training into your daily life.

In Chapter Three, you did a guided fantasy about some scene from your life that ends with your feeling upset. You were supposed to think about your usual reactions and how they affect your body. The method we are going to consider here also uses guided fantasy. It could help you learn better management of your stress and it could help you transfer what you have learned into your daily living. This new method will also be important groundwork to help you learn more about the ideas you use to upset yourself. That will be covered in Part Three of this book.

The method we are talking about involves imagination and its images. Images can be pictures we visualize in our minds, or they can be memories of sounds, or smells, or tastes, or feelings. Usually, images combine memories. When we use our imagination to recreate scenes from past experiences, we can even feel the feelings we had. If the feelings were fun, we can enjoy remembering. If the feelings were unfun, we can stress ourselves again by thinking about them. (Remember how you felt when you imagined yourself in your bad scene? You may have experienced some stress even though you weren't in danger.)

It is possible for you to learn to disconnect some of your upset feelings by using your imagination. One name for this is "desensitization." You can learn to be less sensitive to the things in your life that you feel have caused stress for you. ,

An example of desensitization comes from the wisdom of the Indians of northern California. They developed a method of making themselves less sensitive to poison oak. They had their children rub small pieces of poison oak leaves between their fingers for a short time each day. (This is a little like allergy desensitization treatments that we use today.) Over a period of time, the children became less sensitive to their continual exposure to poison oak. They were desensitized to poison oak.

You can learn to desensitize yourself to things that you believe upset you emotionally. First, get yourself as relaxed as you can by using the methods outlined in Chapter Six of this book. When you are relaxed, imagine yourself in situations that you believe bother you. Keep yourself as relaxed as you can. Imagine yourself being relaxed instead of tense. Now, as you think about yourself being relaxed in your scene, stay relaxed. If you begin to feel upset while you're thinking about your scene, switch your thoughts to relaxing and thinking about your breathing. You know that you can control your stress reactions when you keep your muscles relaxed. You also know that you can think about more than one thing at a time. In this exercise, you imagine being relaxed in your scene while you keep your body relaxed.

This may sound simple, but it will take practice and concentration. It is possible for most people to learn to reduce their stress reactions to some extent in this manner. It is possible — not necessarily easy. When you are doing this, you are transferring your relaxation training into your daily life. Try it. Do it for five or ten minutes each time you do your relaxation exercise. Keep track of your reactions and see if you notice any change.

Here is an example of desensitization. It's about Helen (not her real name, of course). Helen used these methods to learn to manage the upset she felt about high places.

Helen was a well-trained person with a profession. She had trouble working at her profession because she was afraid of heights. She wouldn't go above the ground floor in buildings. Her job involved interviewing people, and the people she wanted to talk to often had offices that were higher than ground floors.

Helen started doing the relaxation exercises twice a day. She did them regularly for two weeks. She learned to get her muscles deeply relaxed and her mind focused on her breathing. She then added some things to her relaxation exercises. She started picturing buildings in her mind. At first she thought about two-story buildings. When she visualized the buildings, she kept her body relaxed. When she felt herself tensing, she went back to thinking about her breathing until she relaxed again.

Gradually, Helen got to the point where she could think of higher buildings. Then she thought about herself standing on the ground looking up at the buildings. With each new step, she would practice until she could think about what she was doing and stay relaxed while she was thinking. She got to where she could imagine going into the buildings and looking at the stairs. After doing this for a while, she decided that in her imagination she would go up one more step each time she did the exercise. She knew that she could stop anywhere and relax, or even come back down the stairs in her imagination.

After two weeks of imagination exercises, Helen was less tense as she thought about high buildings. She stayed relaxed and she cut down the subconscious habit of sending false alarms to her stress system every time she thought about high buildings. The next step was to transfer her training into real life. She started going to buildings and looking up. Then she went into some buildings and looked at some stairs. She started taking one step up each time she went into a building. When she did this, she knew that she could stop and relax herself anytime she wanted to. That way, she was desensitizing herself to the things she had been stressing herself about in the past. Helen kept on with her relaxation each day and she tried to stay as relaxed as she could while she was practicing in the building. She was keeping a log of her success and she was writing down some of the things that went through her mind as she was practicing. (Knowing some of these ideas helped her use the methods in Part Three of this book to correct her errors in thinking about herself and high places.)

Helen learned to manage her stress reaction by using her imagination. In doing so, she gradually developed a new image of herself — an image of more self-confidence. She stopped zapping herself with tiger juice when there weren't any tigers on the stairs or in the elevators. You can do the same thing.

Think about some of the scenes from your life that you think cause you to be upset. Make a list of some of these scenes. Better yet, write a few notes about each scene on small cards. After you have notes on each scene, sort the cards. Put the scene that bothers you the most on top. Rate the other scenes and put them in order going down to the scene that causes the least amount of upset.

After you have your cards sorted, go through them again and check for real danger. Learn to tell the difference between physical danger and psychological danger. Physical danger is a threat to your body. Psychological danger is a threat to your self-image. When you feel a threat to your self-image, you can stress yourself in the same way you would if your *body* was in danger. When you do stress yourself when your body is not in danger, you are stressing yourself in error.

Now, start with the card at the bottom — the one that involves the least stress. Get yourself relaxed. Concentrate on your breathing. Slow down your stress system. When you are relaxed, start imagining yourself in the scene. You are the director, the performers, the audience, and the author. Think about the scene. Really get with it. While you are thinking, *keep your muscles relaxed*. If you find tension building up, go back to concentrating on relaxing and breathing. Do this during your relaxation exercises each day. It won't take a lot of time and it could be very helpful to you.

After you have worked with one scene until you have good control over your stress, try relaxing in the scene *live*. Keep practicing with your imagination, but do some live work also. Make notes on your success and watch for increased efficiency in stress management. As you succeed with one scene, move on to the next harder one in your stack of cards. Keep going until you run out of cards. Remember, you are transferring your skills to real life. You are desensitizing yourself to the things you have upset yourself about in the past. Keep track of the ideas that come to your mind while you are doing this. You can use these ideas as you go on in Part Three of this book to learn to correct your errors in signaling at their source — in your thinking.

Part Three

Stress of Stress Starts In Your Thinking And Can End There Too

11

Thoughts as Errors in Signaling

Do you remember the saying, "Sticks and stones can break my bones, but names can never harm me!"? Do you believe this simple bit of wisdom? Maybe you believe, as many people do, that names *can* harm you. If you believe that names can harm you, you may stress yourself far more than you need to. You may be overly defensive and sensitive, and you probably take things personally.

As you read this, you may be saying, "But I have a right to defend myself when people call me names!" True, you do have that right, but what are you going to defend, and how? Will you be defending your body? Do you have to fight or flee to defend yourself? Could it be that it is your image that you will be defending when people call you names? If so, how much stress energy will you need? Think about it — you could be wasting tiger juice.

Most of us don't fight or run when people call us names. Many of us do *think* ourselves into feeling very uncomfortable though. We really do get ourselves ready to defend our bodies when all that is in danger is what we think of ourselves — our self-images.

It is clear that people who call us unpleasant names probably don't think good things about us, but they can't *think* us into feeling uncomfortable. We do that ourselves. When they call us a name, we think something to ourselves about being called a name. Then we upset ourselves.

If they called us a name in a language we didn't understand, we might not get upset. Even if we understood the language, we would still have to think something before we could upset ourselves.

If another human being started hitting you with sticks or stones it would hurt. It could even kill you. Try to imagine someone hitting you with sticks and stones. Think about how your body would feel. Think what your stress system would be doing. You see, if it were happening, you would need extra energy to run and save your life or to fight if you were in a corner and couldn't run. You would need your stress system to defend yourself.

If another human being started calling you some of your unfavorite names, you might feel unhappy. You might even be angry. You could program stress even if you were certain the person wasn't going to hit you with sticks or stones. You might feel like defending yourself, and waste a lot of stress energy. Again, what would you be defending? Remember, you are reasonably sure that the person isn't going to attack your body. Could it be that your image is under attack? Your hypothalamus doesn't know the difference between your body and your image. It could trigger stress in error. In this way, you would be thinking yourself into an unnecessary stress reaction. Your errors in thinking would be causing discomfort.

Most of our errors in signaling come from our thoughts—the thoughts we have about ourselves, and the things we tell ourselves about our lives. If we convince ourselves that unpleasant things or scenes are dangerous, our errors in signaling can cause us to overreact. (Remember what Epictetus said, "People are not upset by things, but by their ideas about things.")

Other people have written about the way we think ourselves into trouble with our feelings and our actions. Here are a few examples.

"There is nothing either good or bad, but thinking makes it so." (William Shakespeare.)

"Our life is what our thoughts make it." (Marcus Aurelius.)

"Man is the artificer of his own happiness." (Henry David Thoreau.)

"The ancestor of every action is a thought." (Ralph Waldo Emerson.)

"As Thou hast believed, so be it done unto Thee." (Matthew 8:13.)

"Emotion, which is suffering, ceases to be suffering as soon as we form a clear and precise picture of it." (Baruch Spinoza.)

Dr. Albert Ellis (8) is another person who has done a lot to show us how our errors in thinking can cause us trouble. Dr. Ellis has developed a method of helping people think more rationally and stop zapping themselves with unpleasant feelings. This method, which is known as *Rational Emotive Therapy*, uses what Dr. Ellis calls "The A-B-Cs of thinking" to illustrate the way that many of us *think* ourselves into emotional overreactions.

"A" is an *activating* event. Activating events can be tigers, but most of the time they are not. They usually involve communication with other people.

"B" stands for our *beliefs* — the things we tell ourselves about activating events. Our belief systems are usually involved in errors of internal signaling that cause us to think ourselves into being upset.

"C" stands for *consequence*. Consequences can be feelings or behavior. When we are upset, the consequences are usually unpleasant.

Dr. Ellis found that many people believed the unpleasant consequences they experienced were *caused* by activating events ("A"s). His system of helping people involves teaching them to listen to their self-talk at "B" so they will understand the part their thinking plays in their reactions and behavior — the consequences ("C") they experience.

Remember Helen? She was the woman in Chapter Ten with fear of high places. At first, she thought that high places caused her fear. High places were her "A"s and her fears were her "C"s. As she desensitized herself to her fears, she kept track of what she thought to herself when she was around high places. That way, she learned that her beliefs about high places were the main cause of her fears. When she learned to relax around high places, she improved the management of her stress reaction. When she reorganized her thinking about high places, she stopped making errors in thinking that caused her to zap herself with too much tiger juice in the first place.

Our thoughts do influence our emotions and our behavior. We see, we think, and *then* we feel, act, or react.

In some ways it is simple. In some ways it is not. When we take a look at our thinking apparatus, it becomes more complex. For example, we have different levels of thinking, and, we have varying degrees of awareness of our own thoughts. In other words, we do have parts of our minds that are subconscious. In addition, the subconscious parts of our minds can start our stress reactions going. We can have stress of stress and not even know it. Unfortunately, the ideas we have in the subconscious parts of our minds can also trigger our stress reactions in error.

When I use the term "subconscious," I'm talking about ideas and memories that are in the back of my mind — sometimes just out of reach. I'm talking about the subconscious part of my mind when I say, "Her name slips my mind for the moment," or, "I had that word on the tip of my tongue and now it's gone," or, "That idea just came to my mind from nowhere."

If you doubt that you have a subconscious part of your mind, think about this. You have about ten billion brain cells packed into your head. These cells have ways of storing information and of talking to each other about that information. Scientists think that the cells communicate by electrical and chemical signals. They don't know for sure if each brain cell has a way of communicating with every other cell, but a lot of cells do hook up with each other in some way. There is no way that all of the cells could talk about everything they know, all at the same time. There has to be a focus of attention. If all the information in your head got dumped into conscious awareness at the same time, your mind would be blown. You have to have a subconscious part of your mind to survive.

In comparison, think about telephones. There are over four hundred million telephones in the world. Just suppose that everyone who had a telephone was hooked up and talking at the same time. That would be some conference call! If everyone tried to talk at the same time it would surely "blow" something. There would have to be a focus of attention and a lot of people would have to be "on hold." And remember, we're talking about only four hundred million telephones. There are ten *billion* brain cells!

I believe there is a "back of the mind" where ideas are "on hold." I also believe that some of these ideas can send false-alarm messages to the more primitive part of the brain that starts our stress systems going. I believe that the subconscious part of our minds can make errors and start tiger juice going when there aren't any tigers.

If you want to learn more about your "ABC"s of thinking, read *A New Guide to Rational Living*, by Dr. Albert Ellis and Dr. Robert A. Harper (9). If you want to learn more about your brain, read *Mind and Supermind*, edited by Albert Rosenfeld (22).

12

Common Errors in Thinking

In the many years that I have been helping people learn better stress management, I have come to the conclusion that there are errors in thinking that are common to most of us — errors that seem to be built right into the foundations of our culture. I am not the first person to come to this conclusion. Karen Horney (13), Alfred Korzybski (15), and Albert Ellis (8), among others, have been saying this for many years.

In this chapter, I will outline some of the nutty ideas a lot of us have had — ideas that are quite capable of triggering stress in error. They don't have much to do with tigers, but lots to do with tiger juice. In the next chapter I will outline some methods you can use to correct your errors in thinking.

Either/Or Errors in Thinking

How do you rate things? Do you ever catch yourself using terms such as *good* or *bad*? How about *right* or *wrong*? Maybe *fit* or *unfit*? When you rate things this way, you are using either/or thinking. That means you sort things in two piles. You have a two-value system of judgment.

Refer to p. 80

Some people call two-value rating systems "dichotomous reasoning" — I call it "yuck-bucket thinking." I call it that when I catch myself trying to be a perfectionist. When I'm using either/or thinking and sorting things into two buckets, I find that one bucket is marked "perfect," and the other is marked "yuck." When I am doing this, most things go in the yuck bucket. It is hard to be a master perfectionist and get much in the perfect bucket.

It's bad enough when we rate *things* with either/or thinking. It's much more of a problem when we rate *people* that way. Most of us do this — especially when we rate ourselves. You see, when I put myself in the yuck bucket, I move from *feeling* yucky to thinking I *am* yucky. That can be scary when I stop to think about it. Even if I don't stop to think about it consciously, I can scare myself enough to get a lot of tiger juice flowing. Being yucky isn't too far from being inferior or inadequate. Being yucky can be hard on the self-image. I can get scared or mad thinking about it. Either way, I'm wasting precious stress energy. Then I get scared of being scared or mad at being mad and I'm into the vicious cycle of stress of stress. Yuck!

Generalizing Errors in Thinking

When we are in the business of rating things, which a lot of us are, we can go rapidly from a detail to a whole—most of the time without knowing it. For example, if I fail to pass a test, I can say to myself, "I failed to pass the test." That is a detail. If I go on to say, "Therefore, I am a failure," that is a whole. That is also a generalization — an overgeneralization to be exact. After all, if I fail a test in ping-pong, it doesn't automatically follow that I will fail a test in arithmetic. And even if I failed both, it doesn't prove I am a failure as a human being.

In some ways it is as hard to define the word "failure" as it is to define the word "perfect." Lots of people go around getting in trouble with their stress reactions by overgeneralizing in this way. Overgeneralizing a small failure into a larger one can scare the hypothalamus into thinking it's going to be part of the tiger's lunch. When that happens, the hypothalamus seldom fails to start tiger juice flowing.

Absolutistic Errors in Thinking

Do you ever catch yourself using words such as *should, must, have to, always,* or *ought?* These words deal with absolute certainties. If you are using the words very often, you may be subconsciously thinking yourself into unnecessary emotional upsets. You may be stressing yourself in error.

If I say to myself, "I must have success to survive," I am setting myself up for emotional pain, not to mention ulcers, high blood pressure, and other hazards. I am making a vague term, "success," into an absolute necessity for the continuation of my life. If I am saying, "I must have success in outrunning the tiger in order to go on living," it makes sense to stress myself enough to stay alive. A very strong stress reaction to help me escape tigers can save my life. A very strong stress reaction to help me pursue "success" can end my life, or at least make it miserable.

The use of absolutes such as "must" and "should," along with vague terms such as "success" and "glory," can lead to errors in thinking — errors that start stress reactions and waste emergency energy. For example, a bank executive with whom I worked equated "success" with "wealth." His self-talk went something like this, "I must be successful in order to be accepted. To be successful, I must have wealth. It will be horrible if I am not successful." In spite of the fact that he worked with money all of the time, he did not have a clear definition of "wealth." To him the term was like a carrot on a stick — always out of reach no matter how much money he acquired. With this framework, he berated himself for not "succeeding." He was using either/or reasoning (success/failure), along with absolutes (must and should), and he was overgeneralizing ("If I fail to have wealth, I am a failure"). His hypothalamus read this self-talk as an immediate emergency (tigers) and gave him an overload of stress energy (tiger juice). As a final result, he had high blood pressure and chronic neck pain. (His errors in thinking really were "a pain in the neck.")

"Number One" Errors in Thinking

"We're number one. We're number one." How many times have you heard that chant? It happens at sports events. It happens in commercials. Sometimes it seems like an obsession in our culture.

Trying to be as good as possible is fine. Even trying to win and to be "number one" can be great — providing that such striving is not combined with either/or reasoning or overgeneralizing. When the two thoughts are combined, stress energy can be triggered in error.

As an example, I once heard a football coach say, "There is no such thing as second place. There are winners and there are losers."

This coach was using two buckets to sort people. He was also going from details (games won or lost) to wholes (winners and losers). Unfortunately, the coach used the same thinking to judge himself, and he found himself in the yuck bucket more often than he liked. When he did, he stressed himself in error and had many physical problems as a result.

I once worked with an excellent baseball player. I'll call him Charlie since that is not his name. Charlie kept track of the batting averages of all of the baseball players in a four-county area. He rated them on a list that went from the player with the best batting average to the player with the poorest batting average. He was in the fourth place on this list most of the time. When he thought like the coach, he labeled himself as a loser and put himself in the yuck bucket.

Charlie's thinking went something like this. First he rated himself as fourth — on a list that included more than two hundred young men. He then concluded that he was not "number one" (which was a correct observation). Then he made some big errors in thinking. He said to himself, "I am number four. Therefore, I am a loser. I am nothing. I am a zero." He rated himself either/or and went from fourth place on a list of over two hundred to a position that was less than one. He then rated himself as a total failure and gave himself a "global rating." In counseling, we figured out that when Charlie rated himself a zero, his hypothalamus read this as a danger signal. Charlie scared this part of his brain into thinking that his very existence was in danger. His hypothalamus in turn went into action to save Charlie's body, when all that was in danger was his image. As a result of errors in thinking and errors in signaling, Charlie zapped himself with enough tiger juice to start ulcers in his stomach.

In the course of counseling, Charlie developed a more realistic method of rating his skills. He stopped overgeneralizing and he corrected his errors in thinking. He began conserving his stress energy, and his digestive system went back to normal.

"Having Your Cake" Errors

To paraphrase an old saying, "You can't have your cake and eat it too." It applies to much more than cake and most of the time it is true.

In recent years there has been an emphasis on "now." Many people put off important things in their lives in the belief that "Now is the only time we live." They also believe that "The past is gone, the future isn't here yet, so *now* is the time."

As a result of this type of thinking, many people do concentrate on having fun today. Many of them also end up with stress when the future catches them unaware.

The reverse of this old saying can also be stressful. Some people end up with stale cake and stress themselves for that. Both extremes represent errors in thinking that can rob us of emergency energy.

Evelyn's thinking could be an example of "having your cake" errors. She was deeply involved in the "freedom of speech" movement. She believed that she had the right to say anything she wished, anywhere (and she could back this up with quotes from our constitution). She also thought it was terrible that many people rejected her ideas when she spoke freely. Her self-talk included the following, "I have the right to say anything — and they should accept me when I do. It is wrong and terrible when they don't accept me." The primitive part of her brain read her "terrible" as an emergency and prepared her to fight or flee. Since she was determined to "talk," she experienced much more frustration than was healthy for her. She was trying to "eat her cake and have it too" — something that few of us can do.

"Being Different" Errors in Thinking

In our culture we place great emphasis on "equality." Sometimes this emphasis causes confusion — particularly when it goes beyond "equal opportunity." Having equal opportunity is great. Having fear of being "different" is not so great. Some people do expand their strivings for equality into strong fears of being different. When this happens, they stress themselves unnecessarily. They waste stress energy. Then they think that their stress reactions are making them even more different and they suffer from stress of stress — a vicious cycle.

The self-talk for these errors of thinking goes, "I should be like everyone else. What would people think if they knew I was different? That would be horrible!" It is horrible when the penalty for being different is exile into the desert, or having one's head chopped off, or being locked away forever. It is not horrible if we are different and we still have equal opportunity. Society's reaction to "differences" can result in gross injustice and this can lead to inconvenience, sadness, frustration, and many real problems for people. However, stress energy can be wasted when physical fighting or physical running won't help.

John Milton described this type of error in thinking when he said, "It is not miserable to be blind; it is miserable to be incapable of enduring blindness."

Consider errors in thinking. Do you have any? If you do, you can learn some methods of correcting them in the next chapter.

13

How to Correct Your Errors in Thinking

Do you pay attention when you're talking to yourself? Your thoughts are a form of "self-talk," and your thoughts can start your stress going when you don't need it. If you want to cut down on unnecessary stress, try to improve your self-listening skills.

Sometimes you can listen to yourself as you talk. At other times, you can think back over your thoughts later. I call this "INSTANT REPLAY" (2).

To practice instant replay, start keeping track of some of your rough spots and your unpleasant scenes — the things you *think* stress you. Take a few notes, or at least make some mental notes. When you have a few minutes, think back over the scenes. Do an instant replay of the scene as you remember it.

After you have recreated the scene in your mind's eye, go back over the thoughts you had about the scene. Remember the things you were telling yourself about what was going on. Pay special attention to thoughts that trigger stress. Then ask yourself, "Where are the tigers? Was my body really in danger? Did I need extra energy to fight or run?"

When you think back over your reactions, try to separate the physical dangers from the psychological dangers. If your body was in danger, you needed extra energy to defend yourself or to escape. If your self-image was in danger instead of your body, you may have triggered more stress than you needed — this was an error in signaling. Begin to identify these errors. Remember, it is hard to change errors even when you know about them. It is much harder to change them when you don't recognize them. Identify your errors. Then learn to correct them.

Pay special attention to stress that relates to your self-rating. Find out if you are using either/or methods. Find out how often you are rating things about yourself. See if you then go on and overgeneralize about these things and rate *yourself* as a total person. When you find yourself going from a *thing* to a total *self* rating, check to see if you are using either/or reasoning. You are using either/or reasoning when these terms show up: "good" versus "bad;" "adequate" versus "inadequate;" or "yuck" versus "perfect."

Look at the following "Yuck-Bucket Rating Scale." Think about how you have been rating yourself. Self-ratings are important parts of self-images, and self-images are important in stress management.

Read the scale again. Pay special attention to the first and the last categories — "Perfect" and "Yuck." Do you have many *things* about yourself that you rate as perfect? Be honest. If these things are not perfect, are they really yucky? Again, be honest. And last, if the *thing* is yucky, does that make all of *you* yucky? If you are putting all of you in the yuck bucket, you are scaring the older part of your brain. You will manage your stress energies much more efficiently if you improve your thinking in the way you rate yourself.

YUCK-BUCKET RATING SCALE

PERFECT —
impeccable; faultless; supreme; flawless; superhuman; superlative; ultimate.

SUPERIOR —
A; excellent; top-drawer; premium; first-rate; great; exceptional; outstanding.

COMPETENT —
B; meritorious; worthy; valuable; useful; worthwhile; capable; important; esteemed; deserving.

AVERAGE —
C; so-so; medium; ordinary; sufficient; fair; satisfactory.

POOR —
D; tolerable; passing; acceptable; endurable.

INFERIOR —
F; faulty; failing; defective; inadequate; deficient; subordinate; lousy.

YUCK —
hideous; dreadful; horrible; appalling; frightful; horrendous; abominable; revolting; loathsome; detestable; disastrous; ruinous; dire; catastrophic.

Self-inventory Rating Scale

Work up a rating scale — one that has more than two categories. Use the "Yuck-Bucket" scale, or develop one with your favorite and unfavorite words. Just be sure that it has several divisions.

Now take a piece of paper or a notebook and make a list of things about yourself that you like and dislike (this will be a two-bucket sorting to start with, but it may help you see how you have been rating yourself). No one but you has to see the list, so be honest with yourself.

After you have your inventory list, try rating some of the items on the scale you made (or the Yuck-Bucket Rating Scale if you wish).

You may discover that when you rate something about yourself, you consider it in relation to other things. For example, let's suppose that you are six feet six and one of the *things* on your list is height. To give height a rating, you consider it in relation to other factors. If you want to be a basketball player, your height will be at the positive end of the scale. If you want to be a jockey, you are in trouble.

As you can see, ratings are relative. They are comparisons. They are arbitrary. They are not absolute and they don't have to be either/or. They relate to functions. And remember, you are rating *things* about yourself. You are not rating yourself as a total human being.

The more things you rate with your new system, the more you will see the futility of trying to rate yourself as a total person. When you learn that fact at the gut level, your guts will not be bothered as much with unnecessary tiger juice.

Emotions and self-ratings are important when it comes to stress. How you feel about yourself can determine how much you stress yourself. When you rate yourself, keep in mind what Reinhold Niebuhr wrote. He said, "God, grant me the serenity to accept the things I cannot change, the courage to change the things I can, and the wisdom to know the difference."

With Niebuhr's thought in mind, think about your self-image. What are the things you can change? What are the things you cannot change? What do you tell yourself about these things? Listen carefully to your self-talk as you consider these ideas. Your self-talk is an important part of your self-image. Are you being accepting of yourself as a person as you consider things about yourself?

Pick an item on your self-inventory list that you don't like and can't change. Do a relaxation exercise. Think about accepting yourself as a person in spite of the fact that you have this characteristic or this *thing*. Learn to stay relaxed as you think about accepting yourself in this way. Learn to manage your stress and save your energy to change the things you *can* change.

Now pick an item on your inventory that you can change. How would you like to change this part of you? What will you have to do? What are the risks? Do another relaxation exercise. Imagine yourself starting to do some of the important things to bring this change about. Imagine taking the risks involved. Imagine practicing the changes. Consider the ideas that come to mind — excuses you may use to get out of doing what you know is important for you. Using this imagery rehearsal method, you can learn to set your stress system at a level that allows for more efficiency.

As you relax and think of ways you can improve the part of you you have selected, consider options. Imagine trying different approaches. As you think of options, speculate about consequences. See how often you expect the worst. Consider what the real dangers are, particularly the physical dangers. Practice separating dangers to your body from dangers to your image. Reserve your stress energy for dangers to your body.

If you continue to think mainly of catastrophes, deliberately think of some pleasant consequences that you want. Use these to help motivate you, to inspire and to keep you going. Consequences are also relative. A long time ago, Robert G. Ingersoll said, "In nature there are neither rewards nor punishments — there are only consequences."

When you stay relaxed and rehearse the steps necessary to improve the part of you you have selected, start taking the steps *live*. Keep track of what actually happens when you do. Do instant replays of your thinking and your actions and your reactions. Rate your progress with your new rating system. If you practice live, you will begin to transfer your relaxed stress management to your life in general. If you do instant replays, you will have a method of monitoring your thinking — and of reducing errors in thinking that waste stress energy.

Wants Versus Needs

Check your instant replays to see how often you mistake *wants* for *needs*. Ask yourself, "Is this something I really need in order to stay alive?" Pay attention to your answers, especially the times you start your stress reactions going. How much stress energy are you using? How much stress energy are you wasting?

It is natural to want pleasure. It is foolish to zap yourself with as much stress energy for unmet wants as you would for unmet needs (air, water, food, and so forth). Save your tiger juice for tigers.

Try this guided fantasy. Imagine that someone is choking you. Imagine yourself starting to gasp for air. Think what you would do. Think how you would feel. You know you have to have air to live. How hard would you fight to survive?

If you were being choked, you would get some added energy from your stress system. You might need that in order to keep getting the air you also need to survive.

Now think of something you cherish and *want* to keep. Imagine that someone is taking it away from you. Does thinking about this start any of the same reactions you had when you thought about being choked? Compare your reactions. Ask yourself these questions: "Is my life at stake if I don't have what I want? Will I die if I don't have this want? How much stress energy will it take to protect my body if I don't have what I want?"

If you are mistaking wants for needs, you may be wasting stress energy. Learn to separate wants and needs. Use the question, "Will I die if I don't have what I want?" Learn to set your stress reaction where you want it for wants and where you need it for needs. Use relaxation and imagery rehearsal to practice managing your stress energies in these instances. Use instant replay to correct the errors that you can identify in your thinking. With these two methods, you can improve the management of your stress energies. You can survive with less stress of stress.

Correcting Image Errors

Check your instant replays for concerns you have about what you think other people think of you. Ask yourself, "Is my body in danger from sticks and stones (and tigers)? Is my image in danger from names that are not supposed to harm me?" If you find that you are programming enough stress to protect your body when it is your image that is in danger, try these methods to improve your errors in signaling and your errors in thinking. Practice relaxation and think about people calling you names and thinking unpleasant thoughts about you. Try to stay relaxed and manage your stress reactions. Remember Helen in Chapter Ten? Remember that she thought about high places and stayed relaxed. Then she practiced going to high places and staying relaxed. Then she stayed relaxed and considered some of the things she thought to herself about her own self-image.

Practice imagining yourself in situations where people do have negative thoughts about you. Stay as relaxed as you can while you think about doing this. Imagine yourself being in such situations and not overreacting. Remember, I am not suggesting that you ignore what people say about you or what people think about you. I am suggesting that you learn to manage your stress reaction in such situations so that you will reduce your overreacting and conserve your emergency energies. You can do this more efficiently if you are aware of what it is you may want to defend when people are calling you names. It does not take the same amount of energy to defend your image as it does to defend your body. Also, keep in mind that if you have a realistic method of rating things about yourself, you will feel less vulnerable when other people are rating you. When you practice staying relaxed as you think about these things in instant replay, you are desensitizing yourself to your stressors. You are correcting your errors in signaling and your errors in thinking.

How to Correct Errors in
Thinking About Being Different

Have you ever been to a masquerade party? I worked with a very successful businessman once who said to me, "I have to go to a masquerade party next Halloween and I'm tempted to go disguised as my *true* self." Naturally, I listened further.

This man appeared to have all the things most of us strive for. He had money, social position, economic power, prestige, and a beautiful family. He was not happy, however, and he frequently talked about having to "play a role." He felt that deep down he was really quite different from most people. He often said, "What would people think of me if they knew how different I was?"

After listening to him, I suggested that he consider taking some risk by going to the party "disguised" as his true self. We had several weeks to work so he began to define the ways in which he felt he was different. After he had his character (and his costume) worked up, he started relaxing and rehearsing going to the party as "himself."

He considered some of the reactions he would get from other people. He also thought about what he would be saying to himself about some of the reactions he expected. As he did this rehearsing, he tried to keep his stress reactions within reasonable limits by relaxation.

As it turned out, he went as his "true self" and he also wore a sign around his neck that read, "This is the real me! So what?"

It was a successful experiment. He was a hit! He shared his differences with his peers and he found that the "So what?" wasn't as stressful as he had always thought it would be.

You can try something like this yourself. (If you are not going to be attending a masquerade party, I would suggest that you do it without a sign.)

Think about the ways in which you are different. Do you try to *hide* these differences? Consider sharing your differences more openly — without self-blame and with an open mind to the feedback you may get. Anticipate the self-talk you will be doing. Try to correct your errors in thinking as you stay relaxed. Practice relaxing as you plan your approach.

Take your differences one at a time. Keep track of the results. You may find you have been programming yourself to use much more stress energy than you need. Who knows, you might even begin to accept yourself as you see yourself! If you do, your hypothalamus will stop making you as defensive about your "image." You may even get to be one of your own best friends. If you do, you will cut down on your stress of stress.

How to Correct Errors in Thinking
That Lead to Procrastination

Procrastination is easy for some of us. Sometimes the *results* of procrastination are not easy to live with. Procrastination can stem from errors in thinking, when you fool yourself into believing that you can "have your cake and eat it too." You may tell yourself you can have your pleasure today and still have it in all of your tomorrows. Sometimes you can. Most of the time you can't.

Here's how to correct your errors in thinking about procrastination. Keep track of your emotional upsets that relate to procrastination. Relax and do instant replays about the situations involved. Figure out what decisions you made and when you made them. Try to recall what your self-talk was just before you made the decisions. Look for times when you fooled yourself into thinking you could have your cake and eat it too, or said to yourself, "I can have my pleasure *now* and have it again tomorrow." Pay special attention to times when tomorrow's pleasures may depend on hard work done today.

When you start pinpointing your decisions, you will be better at identifying the consequences of your decisions. If the consequences result in unnecessary stress, you may want to change some of your decisions.

Try this experiment. Set a goal for yourself. At first, try a simple goal with short time limits. For instance, "I want to have all my extra work done by next weekend so I can have some time to do whatever I want." Keep this goal in mind. When you catch yourself loafing or goofing off, ask yourself, "How will this ten minutes of loafing affect my goal?" Try to identify the times you kid yourself by saying, "I can loaf now and still have everything done by the weekend." Maybe you can. Then again, maybe you can't.

You can also try another experiment. After you finish doing your relaxation and meditation, spend a few minutes thinking about the fun things you can do on your weekend. When you have this pleasure goal well in mind, it will make it easier to keep yourself from procrastinating between now and next weekend. That way, you will cut down on the stress that procrastination can be causing you.

After you succeed with a simple goal, pick a larger one. Use the same technique. By combining short-term goals with long-term goals, you could end up having some fun today and some fun tomorrow. That's as close as most of us will come to "having our cake and eating it too."

You now have some ways to help you improve your stress management. You have not found instant happiness nor have you found a "cure-all" for the ailments of the world. You have learned that your stress reaction is a natural part of being human. You have read about specific ways you can use to conserve and manage your stress energy. If you relax and meditate, you can correct your errors in signaling that waste energy. If you learn to listen to your self-talk, you can correct some of your errors in thinking that cause trouble for you to begin with. Use the exercises. Practice. Practice. Practice. You could live longer and have more fun while you're living!

In this book I have emphasized methods of stress management. I have not gone into detail about the multitude of "things" that serve as stressors for people. In the next chapter I will describe some things that can serve as stressors. The list does not include all things that have served as stressors for people. I don't know of any list that complete.

Epilogue

14
Other Stressors of Life

"Emotion, which is suffering, ceases to be suffering as soon as we form a clear and precise picture of it." (Baruch Spinoza.)

This chapter will describe some stressors we can encounter that are hard to change — stressors that are sometimes hard to even identify. As Spinoza points out, emotional suffering can be reduced if identified. Learning to identify stressors will at least give you a better idea of what you can and cannot do about them.

Most of this book has been about ways you can manage your stress reaction as you adapt to your world as it is. Some of the stressors described in this chapter may require environmental changes for reduction in emotional suffering. If you have tried all of the stress management methods described so far, and you are still suffering emotional pain, you may need to improve your methods of identification of stressors and make some changes in your life patterns or your environment.

In Chapter Thirteen I included Reinhold Niebuhr's famous saying, "God, grant me the serenity to accept the things I cannot change, the courage to change the things I can, and the wisdom to know the difference." You may have tried the self-inventory and the relaxation and desensitization exercises to put Niebuhr's philosophy into action. If you were successful, that is great. If you were not, you may want to consider some of the following ideas.

Two factors to consider in relation to stressors are: how hard are they to identify; and, how hard are they to change after they are identified.

Identification of Hard to Change Stressors

Stressors can range all the way from "mini" to "maxi," and both can trigger stress reactions. A mini-stressor could be subliminal (just below conscious awareness) and it could be just barely noticeable. A maxi-stressor would be one that was quite obvious. For example, take noise. A mini-stressor involving noise could be a sound intensity that was quite low, such as the slight humming of a machine. A maxi-stressor could be the banging and clanging of a boiler room or the roar of traffic.

You could be having some stress reaction from either of these intensities of noise and it is possible that you wouldn't know about it — the stress reaction, that is. Stimulation of our senses can result in this type of problem. For example, some people can become agitated by various types of light fixtures. They can be agitated and not know the source of their agitation. It is even possible to have a combination of low-level, sensory stimulation that triggers stress reactions. If you work day after day in a place that is cold, has constant noise pollution, poor lighting, and noxious smells, the chances are you suffer from excessive stress reaction. Under the circumstances just described, you will be limited in what you can do with the methods described so far in this book to manage your stress reactions. Meditation, exercise, and awareness of your inner thoughts will help, but these methods would not be enough to stop the excessive use of your stress energies. Some environmental change might be necessary if you were to stop jeopardizing your health by the constant triggering of your stress reaction.

The first step in management of this type is identification. Learn to be aware of your environment *and your body's reaction to your environment*. If you can identify stressors, you are in a much better position to decide how far you can go in changing them.

Duration of exposure to stressors is also important. The range here can go from occasional to constant. If you are around loud noise once in a while, it is one thing. If you have to endure constant exposure to loud noise, it is another. In evaluating your stressors, consider both the intensity and the duration. After you have identified your stressors, consider what you can do to make changes in your environment. If the stressors can be changed, change them. If they cannot be changed, you may want to consider how important it is for you to remain in the environment of the stressors.

Milestone Stressors

All of us go through changes as we go through life. Some of us seem to adjust to these changes without much reaction. Some of us have considerable reaction to the various changes. Most of us have *some* stress reaction as we face the prospect of these changes.

Some of the more apparent milestones are: puberty; emancipation from parents; mating; parenting; middle age; climacteric changes (menopause for females); old age; and death.

What we tell ourselves about our ever changing images in relation to milestones can trigger stress reaction. In addition, I believe that the changes themselves can trigger some stress. I believe that Spinoza's thoughts can be helpful here. Knowing the facts involved in these changes can help reduce some of the emotional suffering. To learn about the milestones of development we all go through, read Gail Sheehy's best-selling book, *Passages* (28).

Real Catastrophes

In Chapter Thirteen I described how some of us anticipate catastrophes when we rate ourselves (see Yuck-Bucket Rating Scale on page 87). Self-rating catastrophes are one thing. Real catastrophes are another. Many of us can have the misfortune to experience real catastrophes — accidents, earthquakes, floods, fires, famines, and many more. Such catastrophes do trigger our stress reactions when we experience them. Sometimes we can use emergency energy to help us survive. Sometimes we cannot. (Fighting a tiger takes lots of energy. Fighting a steering wheel on a slippery road does not take that much energy.)

If you are in the middle of a real catastrophe, or if you are recovering from a recent one, it will be hard for you to learn stress management with the methods described in this book. If you learn to use the methods in this book, and practice them, you will be better able to manage your stress if you have the misfortune to experience a catastrophe later on. If you try to learn them after you are in a crisis situation, you will be disappointed to say the least.

Meaning of Life Stress

"He who has a *why* to live can bear with almost any *how*." (Friedrich Nietzsche.)

Many people in the world suffer excessive stress reactions because they are bored. Other people stress themselves because they feel their lives are meaningless.

Sensory deprivation can cause stress-related problems just as sensory "overload" can cause problems. In evaluating your stress management, give consideration to the meaning you place on life. In today's world there are many options open to us in terms of philosophy and religion, or any method of defining the meaning of life.

Dr. Viktor Frankl, in his book, *Man's Search for Meaning* (10), talked about the options open to us when he said, "The last of human freedoms is the ability to choose one's attitude in a given set of circumstances." Dr. Frankl lived through the holocaust of Nazi concentration camps during World War II. He felt that people around him in the concentration camps had better chances of survival if they had some sense of meaning in their lives. When you are evaluating your stress management system, give some thought to the way you look at the meaning of life. You may be overlooking a helpful method of stress management if you have no philosophy of life or no method of sensing the meaning of your life.

Professional Help With
Stress Management

All self-help books have limitations. This book is no exception. We all have blind spots in our methods of looking at ourselves. If you have tried the methods of stress management I have described, and you are still experiencing emotional suffering, you may want to get some professional help. Don't be afraid to at least give the idea of help some thought. (If you are worried about how getting professional help with your emotional problems will affect your "image," you can use the methods of this book to work through that dilemma!)

If you decide to get help, don't hesitate to ask therapists to describe their methods and philosophies. Professionally trained therapists are usually willing to discuss their methods although they don't always do so unless asked. You and the therapist will benefit by a clear definition of what you expect from therapy.

15

A Few Words About What You've Learned

It may be that the 1980s, on Planet Earth, will be known as the time when humans faced the fact that many energy supplies are finite, and therefore limited. If we learn that lesson, and face that fact, we can set about learning better management and conservation of energy. If not, future generations will learn the hard way that when energy is gone, it's gone.

One purpose of this book is to describe emergency energy supplies within all human beings. Human stress energy is a natural resource which may also be finite, and therefore limited. Another purpose of this book has been to describe ways in which we can better manage this energy and conserve this resource.

On earth we live with rapidly developing technology that has provided us with ways to explore our solar system — and maybe to destroy it if we are not careful. In spite of our technology, we still live in bodies that are geared for fleeing and for fighting Saber Tooth Tigers. Even though we have learned to think in scientific ways, we still have many nutty and unscientific ways of thinking about stress. Many people today teach their children that fear is not for males and anger is not for females. Many people believe that the stress reaction is weakness, when it is *really strength.* Many myths about stress exist. This book was designed to help eliminate some of the myths that cause us to trigger our stress in error and waste our emergency energies.

In the first part of this book, I described the natural purposes, functions, and anatomy of stress. In the second part, I outlined methods of physical management of stress through relaxation, meditation, exercise, biofeedback, imagination, and desensitization. In the third part, I showed how many of us think in error and therefore trigger stress in error. I also pointed out that since we think our way into unnecessary stress, we can learn to think our way out. I gave you specific exercises for developing these new ways of thinking.

If you practice the relaxation, meditation, physical exercise, and biofeedback methods, you will have a way of reducing stress when you trigger it in error. If you use your imagination, and desensitize yourself to your stressors you will be able to transfer your stress management skills into your everyday world. If you then practice the new ways of thinking, you can learn to correct stress errors at their source — in your thinking. Combining all these methods, you could learn to conserve your deep emergency energy for its true purpose — to help you survive physical danger. You could also have much more fun using your energies in pleasant and more productive ways.

This book is not a panacea to cure all ailments or to solve all problems. If you use the methods in the book, you can conserve your energies and become more efficient at solving some of the problems you face. You can learn to take charge of your life and assume more responsibility for yourself.

I have not described ways for you to change your outer environment. It may be that a change in environment or life style would be helpful to you in solving some of your problems. By using the methods in this book, you can become more realistic in making decisions regarding your environment and life style.

The methods in this book are simple, but they are not easy. They require practice, practice, practice. To succeed, a commitment on your part will be necessary. You will have to call on your will power if you are going to follow through in improving your life situation and reducing your stress reaction.

If you have tried the methods in this book and you are still experiencing more stress than you want to have, consider getting further help from a professionally trained therapist.

If the book has helped you learn more about yourself and your natural stress reaction, I am glad. If you have developed better stress management and have less stress of stress, you may be glad. If we teach some of these ideas and methods to others — particularly our children — we can all rejoice in the hope that future generations will avoid unnecessary pain and suffering from stress systems that are out of control.

Bibliography

Bibliography

1. Bedford, Stewart, *Instant Replay*. New York: Institute for Rational Living, Inc., 1974.
2. Bedford, Stewart, *Instant Replay: A Method of Counseling Little (and Other) People*. New York: Institute for Rational Living, 1974.
3. Benson, Herbert, *The Relaxation Response*. New York: William Morrow and Co., 1975.
4. Brooke, Avery, *Hidden in Plain Sight: The Practice of Christian Meditation*. New York: The Seabury Press, 1978.
5. Brown, Barbara B., *Stress and the Art of Biofeedback*. New York: Harper and Row, 1977.
6. Cannon, Walter B., *The Wisdom of the Body*. New York: W. W. Norton, 1932.
7. Cooper, Kenneth, *The New Aerobics*. New York: Bantam Books, 1970.
8. Ellis, Albert, *Humanistic Psychotherapy: The Rational-Emotive Approach*. New York: The Julian Press, Inc., 1973.
9. Ellis, Albert, and Harper, Robert A., *A New Guide to Rational Living*. Englewood Cliffs, New Jersey: Prentice Hall, Inc., 1975.
10. Frankl, Viktor E., *Man's Search for Meaning: An Introduction to Logotherapy*. New York: Washington Square Press, Inc., 1963.
11. Goleman, Daniel, *The Varieties of the Meditative Experience*. New York: E. P. Dutton, 1977.

12. Hess, W. R., *The Functional Organization of the Diencephalon.* New York: Grune and Stratton, 1957.

13. Horney, Karen, *The Neurotic Personality of Our Time.* New York: W. W. Norton, 1937.

14. Jacobson, Edmund, *You Must Relax.* New York: McGraw-Hill Book Co., Inc., 1934.

15. Korzybski, Alfred, *Science and Sanity: An Introduction to Non-Aristotelian Systems and General Semantics.* Lancaster, Pa.: The Science Press, 1933.

16. Luthe, Wolfgang, *Autogenic Therapy.* New York: Grune and Stratton, 1969.

17. Maultsby, Maxie C., Jr., and Hendricks, Allie, *You and Your Emotions.* Lexington, Kentucky: University of Kentucky Medical Center, 1974.

18. McQuade, Walter, and Aikman, Ann, *Stress: What It Is; What It Can Do to Your Health; How to Fight Back.* New York: E. P. Dutton and Co., Inc., 1974.

19. Morehouse, Laurence E. and Gross, Leonard, *Total Fitness in 30 Minutes a Week.* New York: Simon and Schuster, Inc., 1975.

20. Naranjo, Claudio, and Ornstein, Robert E., *On the Psychology of Meditation.* New York: The Viking Press, 1971.

21. Pelletier, Kenneth R., *Mind As Healer, Mind As Slayer.* New York: Del Corte Press, 1977.

22. Rosenfeld, Albert, editor, *Mind and Supermind.* New York: Holt, Rinehart and Winston, 1973.

23. Sagan, Carl, *The Dragons of Eden.* New York: Random House, 1977.

24. Samuels, Mike, and Samuels, Nancy, *Seeing with the Mind's Eye: The History, Techniques and Uses of Visualization.* New York: Random House, 1975.

25. Schultz, J. H., and Luthe, Wolfgang, *Autogenic Training: A Psychophysiological Approach to Psychotherapy.* New York: Grune and Stratton, 1959.
26. Schwartz, Gary E., *Biofeedback: Theory and Research.* New York: Academic Press, 1977.
27. Selye, Hans, *Stress Without Distress.* New York: J. B. Lippincott Co., 1974.
28. Sheehy, Gail, *Passages: Predictable Crises of Adult Life.* New York: E. P. Dutton, 1976.
29. Singer, Jerome L., *Imagery and Daydream Methods in Psychotherapy and Behavior Modification.* New York: Academic Press, 1974.
30. Solomon, Neil, and Harrison, Evalee, *Doctor Solomon's Proven Master Plan for Total Body Fitness and Maintenance.* New York: G. P. Putnam's Sons, 1976.
31. Tart, Charles T., *Altered States of Consciousness.* New York: Doubleday & Co., 1969.

Index

Index

118

NOTES

NOTES

NOTES

NOTES

Tapes Available:

Cassette tapes on relaxation and stress management
are available from Scott Publications. The tapes
are written and spoken by Dr. Stewart Bedford,
author of this book.

Write:

Scott
Publications
P.O. Box 3277
Chico, California 95927